AF499281

Contents

What is COPD (chronic obstructive pulmonary disease)?

COPD is an umbrella term for a range of progressive lung diseases. Chronic bronchitis and emphysema both can result in COPD. A COPD diagnosis means you may have one of these lung-damaging diseases or symptoms of both. COPD can progress gradually, making it increasingly difficult to breathe over time.

Chronic bronchitis

Chronic bronchitis irritates your bronchial tubes, which carry air to and from your lungs. In response, the tubes swell and mucus (phlegm or "snot") builds up along the lining. The buildup narrows the tube's opening, making it hard to get air in and out of the lungs.

Small, hair-like structures on the inside of the bronchial tubes (called cilia) normally move mucus out of the airways. But the irritation from chronic bronchitis and/or smoking damages them. The damaged cilia can't help clear mucus.

Emphysema

Emphysema is the breakdown of the walls of the tiny air sacs (alveoli) at the end of the bronchial tubes, in the "bottom" of the lung. The lung is like an upside down tree. The trunk is the windpipe or "trachea," the branches are the "bronchi," and the leaves are the air sacs or "alveoli ." The air sacs play a crucial role in transferring oxygen into your blood and carbon dioxide out. The damage caused by emphysema destroys the walls of the air sacs, making it hard to get a full breath.

How common is COPD?

COPD affects nearly 16 million Americans, or about 6% of the U.S. population.

Who gets COPD?

The primary cause of COPD is smoking. But not all smokers develop the disease. You may be at higher risk if you:

- Are a woman.
- Are over the age of 65.
- Have been exposed to air pollution.
- Have worked with chemicals, dust or fumes.

• Have alpha-1 antitrypsin deficiency (AAT), a genetic risk factor to develop COPD.

• Had many respiratory infections during childhood.

SYMPTOMS AND CAUSES

What causes COPD?

Smoking tobacco causes up to 90% of COPD cases. Other causes include:

• Alpha-1 antitrypsin (AAT) deficiency, a genetic disorder.

• Secondhand smoke.

• Air pollution.

• Workplace dust and fumes.

Smoking

Tobacco smoke irritates airways, triggering inflammation (irritation and swelling) that narrows the airways. Smoke also damages cilia so they can't do their job of removing mucus and trapped particles from the airways.

AAT deficiency

AAT (alpha-1 antitrypsin deficiency) is an uncommon, inherited disorder that can lead to emphysema. Alpha-1 antitrypsin is an enzyme that helps protect lungs from the damaging effects of inflammation. When you have AAT, you don't produce enough of the enzyme, called alpha-1 antitrypsin. Your lungs are more likely to become damaged from exposure to irritating substances like smoke and dust.

What are signs of chronic obstructive pulmonary disease (COPD)?

- Cough with mucus that persists for long periods of time.

- Difficulty taking a deep breath.

- Shortness of breath with mild exercise (like walking or using the stairs).

- Shortness of breath performing regular daily activities.

- Wheezing.

If I am having chronic obstructive pulmonary disease symptoms, how do I determine when I need to call my doctor?

If you are having any of the symptoms described below, don't wait for your next appointment to call your doctor. Report these symptoms promptly, even if you don't feel sick. DO NOT wait for symptoms to become so severe that you need to seek emergency care. If your symptoms are discovered early, your doctor might change your treatment or medications to relieve your symptoms. (Never change or stop taking your medications without first talking to your doctor).

Note: Remember that warning signs or symptoms might be the same or different from one flare-up to another.

Non-emergency care

Talk to your doctor on the phone within 24 hours if you have these changes in your health:

- Shortness of breath that has become worse or occurs more often. Examples:

o Unable to walk as far as usual

o Need more pillows or have to sit up to sleep because of breathing difficulty

o More tired because you're working harder to breathe

o Need breathing treatments or inhalers more often than usual

o Wake up short of breath more than once a night

• Sputum (mucus) changes including:

o Changes in color

o Presence of blood

o Changes in thickness or amount (more than you usually have or more than you are able to cough out)

- Odor

- More coughing or wheezing
- Swelling in your ankles, feet, or legs that is new or has become worse and doesn't go away after a night's sleep with your feet up
- Unexplained weight loss or gain of 2 pounds in a day or 5 pounds in a week
- Frequent morning headaches or dizziness
- Fever, especially with cold or flu symptoms
- Restlessness, confusion, forgetfulness, slurring of speech, or irritability
- Unexplained, extreme fatigue or weakness that lasts for more than a day

DIAGNOSIS AND TESTS

How is chronic obstructive pulmonary disease (COPD) diagnosed?

To assess your lungs and overall health, your healthcare provider will take your medical history, perform a physical exam and order some tests, like breathing tests.

Medical history

To diagnose COPD, your provider will ask questions like:

- Do you smoke?
- Have you had long-term exposure to dust or air pollutants?
- Do other members of your family have COPD?

- Do you get short of breath with exercise? When resting?
- Have you been coughing or wheezing for a long time?
- Do you cough up phlegm?

Physical exam

To help with the diagnosis, your provider will do a physical exam that includes:

- Listening to your lungs and heart.
- Checking your blood pressure and pulse.
- Examining your nose and throat.
- Checking your feet and ankles for swelling.

Tests

Providers use a simple test called spirometry to see how well your lungs work. For this test, you blow air into a tube attached to a machine. This lung function test measures how much air you can breathe out and how fast you can do it.

Your provider may also want to run a few other tests, such as:

- Pulse oximetry to measure the oxygen in your blood.
- Arterial blood gases (ABGs) to check your oxygen and carbon dioxide levels.
- Electrocardiogram (ECG or EKG) to check heart function and rule out heart disease as a cause of shortness of breath.
- Chest X-ray or chest CT scan to look for lung changes that are caused by COPD.

- Exercise testing to determine if the oxygen level in your blood drops when you exercise.

What are the stages of COPD?

COPD can gradually get worse. How fast it progresses from mild to severe varies from person to person.

Mild COPD (stage 1 or early stage)

The first sign of COPD is often feeling out of breath with light exercise, like walking up stairs. Because it's easy to blame this symptom on being out of shape or getting older, many people don't realize they have COPD. Another sign is a phlegmy cough (a cough with mucus) that's often particularly troublesome in the morning.

Moderate to severe COPD (stages 2 and 3)

In general, shortness of breath is more evident with more advanced COPD. You may develop shortness of breath even during everyday activities. Also, exacerbations of COPD – times when you experience increased phlegm, discoloration of phlegm, and more shortness of breath – are generally more common in higher stages of COPD. You also become prone to lung infections like bronchitis and pneumonia.

Very severe COPD (stage 4)

When COPD becomes severe, almost everything you do can cause shortness of breath. This limits your mobility. You may need supplemental oxygen from a portable tank.

MANAGEMENT AND TREATMENT

How is chronic obstructive pulmonary disease (COPD) managed?

COPD treatment focuses on relieving symptoms, such as coughing and breathing problems, and avoiding respiratory infections. Your provider may recommend:

- Bronchodilators: These medicines relax airways. Delivered through a mist you inhale, bronchodilators help you breathe easier.

- Anti-inflammatory medications: Doctors commonly prescribe steroids to lower inflammation in the lungs. You inhale steroids in a mist form (nebulizer or inhaler) or take them by swallowing a pill.

- Supplemental oxygen: If you have low blood oxygen (hypoxemia), you may need a portable oxygen tank to improve your oxygen levels.

- Antibiotics: COPD makes you prone to lung infections, which can further damage your weakened lungs. Your doctor may prescribe antibiotics to stop a bacterial infection.

- Vaccinations: Respiratory infections are more dangerous when you have COPD. It's especially important to get shots to prevent flu and pneumonia.

- Rehabilitation: Rehabilitation programs focus on teaching effective breathing strategies to lessen shortness of breath and on conditioning. When maintained, fitness can increase the amount you can do with the lungs you have.

- Anticholinergics relax the muscle bands that tighten around the airways. This action opens the airways, letting more air in and out of the lungs to improve breathing. Anticholinergics also help clear mucus from the lungs. As the airways open, the mucus moves more freely and can therefore be coughed out more easily. Anticholinergics work differently and more slowly than fast-acting bronchodilators.

- Leukotriene modifiers might be used. Leukotrienes are chemicals that occur naturally in our bodies and cause tightening of airway muscles, and production of mucus and fluid. These newer drugs work by blocking the chemicals and decreasing these reactions. These medications help improve airflow and reduce symptoms in some people.

- Expectorants thin mucus in the airways so it can be coughed out more easily. Take these medications with about 8 ounces of water.

- Antihistamines relieve stuffy heads, watery eyes, and sneezing. Although effective at relieving these symptoms, antihistamines can dry the air passages, making breathing difficult, as well as causing difficulty when coughing up excess mucus. Take these medications with food to reduce upset stomach.

- Antivirals might be prescribed to treat or prevent illnesses caused by viruses, most frequently to treat or prevent influenza ("the flu"). Influenza is particularly dangerous for people who have COPD.

For severe COPD, your provider may suggest you consider a clinical trial (tests of new treatments) or lung surgery, if you're a candidate.

PREVENTION

How can I avoid COPD?

The best thing you can do to avoid developing COPD is to not smoke. If you'd like to quit, smoking cessation programs can help you. Also, avoid any environment that has poor air quality — air that has particles like dust, smoke, gases and fumes.

Why should people with COPD (chronic obstructive pulmonary disease) watch for signs of infection?

People with COPD have difficulty clearing their lungs of bacteria, dusts and other pollutants in the air. This makes them at risk for lung infections that may cause further damage to the lungs.

Therefore, it is important to watch for signs of infection and follow these tips to help prevent infections. You will probably not be able to avoid infections entirely, but these tips will help you prevent infections as much as possible.

What are warning signs of an infection, especially if I have COPD (chronic obstructive pulmonary disease)?

Warning signs of infection

While most infections can be successfully treated, you must be able to recognize an infection's immediate symptoms for proper and effective care.

- Increased shortness of breath, difficulty breathing or wheezing
- Coughing up increased amounts of mucus
- Yellow- or green-colored mucus (may or may not be present)
- Fever (temperature over 101°F) or chills (may or may not be present)

- Increased fatigue or weakness
- Sore throat, scratchy throat or pain when swallowing
- Unusual sinus drainage, nasal congestion, headaches or tenderness along upper cheekbones

If you have any of these symptoms, contact your physician right away, even if you do not feel sick.

What can I do to prevent infections, especially if I have COPD (chronic obstructive pulmonary disease)?

Hand washing

Frequently wash your hands with soap and warm water, especially before preparing food, eating, taking medications or breathing treatments; and after coughing or sneezing, using the bathroom, touching soiled linens or clothes, and after you've been around someone with a cold or the flu as well as after you've been at a social gathering. It is also good to carry waterless hand sanitizers with you to use when necessary.

Visitors

If visitors have cold or flu symptoms, ask them not to visit until they are feeling well.

Environment

- Keep your house clean and free from excess dust. Keep your bathrooms and sinks free from mold or mildew.

- Do not work in or visit any form of construction site. Dust can be harmful. If you absolutely must go near this type of area, wear a mask provided by your doctor.

- Avoid air pollution, including tobacco smoke, wood or oil smoke, car exhaust fumes and industrial pollution which can cause inhaled irritants to enter your lungs. Also avoid pollen.

- Make sure your cooking vent is working properly so cooking fumes can be drawn out of the house.

- If possible, try to stay away from large crowds in the fall and winter when the flu season is at its peak.

Equipment care

- Keep breathing equipment clean.

• Do not let others use your medical equipment, including: oxygen cannula, metered dose inhaler (MDI), MDI spacer, nebulizer tubing and mouthpiece.

Diet

1. Try to eat a balanced diet. Good nutrition is important to help the body resist infection. Eat foods from all the food groups.

2. Drink plenty of fluids—at least 6 to 8 eight-ounce glasses per day (unless your doctor gives you other guidelines). Water, juices and sports drinks are best.

Other general health guidelines

• Do not rub your eyes, as this can transmit germs to your nasal passages via the tear ducts.

- Quitting smoking and avoiding second-hand smoke (the smoke from a burning cigarette or cigar and the smoke exhaled by a smoker) are important steps you can take to protect your lungs from infection.

- Follow your doctor's medication guidelines.

- Get enough sleep and rest.

- Manage your stress.

- Talk to your doctor or healthcare provider about getting a flu shot every year and get the pneumonia vaccine if you have not had one.

- Be careful to avoid infection when traveling. In areas where the water might be unsafe, drink bottled water or other beverages (order beverages without ice). Swim only in chlorinated pools.

OUTLOOK / PROGNOSIS

What is the outlook?

COPD progresses at a different rate for every person. Once it progresses, the lung damage from COPD can't be reversed but, by following a healthy lifestyle and getting treatment as early as possible, you can manage symptoms and feel much better.

LIVING WITH

How can I manage COPD at home?

You can take several steps to make breathing easier and slow the progression of the disease:

- Quit smoking.

- Avoid air polluted by chemicals, smoke, dust or fumes.

- Take prescribed medications as directed by your provider.

- Ask your doctor about a pulmonary rehabilitation program, which teaches you how to be active with less shortness of breath.

- Maintain a healthy weight.

- Get an annual flu shot.

The good news about COPD is that the symptoms can be managed. You'll breathe easier if you take the necessary steps to support your lung capacity and fight lung irritation. By getting treatment early, you'll have the best shot at continuing to do the things you love.

When should I call my doctor if I have COPD (chronic obstructive pulmonary disease) and I might have an infection?

Call your doctor if you experience any of the warning signs of an infection. Also call your doctor if you have any symptoms that cause concern.

Avoiding irritants

The lungs of people with COPD are sensitive to certain irritating substances in the air, such as: cigarette smoke, exhaust fumes, strong perfumes, cleaning products, paint/varnish, dust, pollen, pet dander and air pollution. Extreme cold or hot weather conditions can also irritate your lungs.

You can avoid some of these irritants by:

- Asking those around you not to smoke.
- Sitting in non-smoking sections of public places.
- Requesting smoke-free hotel rooms and rental cars.
- Avoiding underground parking garages.
- Avoiding high traffic or industrialized areas.
- Not using perfumes, scented lotions or other highly scented products that may irritate your lungs.
- Using non-aerosol cleaning or painting products in well-ventilated areas and wearing a mask or handkerchief over your mouth when cleaning (dusting, vacuuming, sweeping) or working in the yard.

- Reducing exposure to dust by regularly changing filters on heaters and air conditioners and using a dehumidifier.

- Keeping pets out of the house, especially if you wheeze.

- Using an exhaust fan when cooking to remove smoke and odors.

- Staying indoors when the outside air quality is poor and pollen counts are high.

- Following weather reports and avoiding extreme weather. During cold weather, cover your face when going outdoors. During extreme humidity, try to stay in air conditioned areas.

How does COPD affect the body?

COPD can lead to changes in a person's metabolism and body composition.

Changes in metabolism

Metabolism is the process that occurs within the body to sustain life, such as converting the food a person eats into energy.

According to an article in The Journal of Translational Medicine, many people with COPD are in a state of hyper-metabolism. This is where the body uses more energy to perform essential body functions, such as breathing.

A person who has COPD and hyper-metabolism will require more calories than someone who does not have these conditions.

Changes in body composition

Around 25-40% of people with COPD develop pulmonary cachexia syndrome (PCS). This is a metabolic condition that causes weight loss and muscle wasting.

Some factors that may contribute to PCS in COPD include:

- widespread, or systemic, inflammation
- hyper-metabolism and insufficient calorie intake
- increased energy expenditure due to more effortful breathing
- muscle atrophy resulting from inactivity
- use of glucocorticoid medications to treat COPD

People with COPD and PCS typically require dietary interventions to counteract the PCS and prevent further health complications.

COPD and weight

People with COPD who have underweight or overweight may encounter additional health issues.

Being underweight can sometimes indicate malnutrition. A 2019 review notes that malnutrition alongside COPD may lead to poor health outcomes, including increased risk of COPD exacerbations or flare-ups.

According to a 2013 review, people who have COPD with obesity tend to experience more significant breathing difficulties compared to people with COPD without obesity. According to the review, excess fat, or adipose tissue, puts pressure on the chest wall, exacerbating breathing difficulties.

A 2014 review suggests that controlling obesity may help prevent and manage lung impairment in people with COPD.

If a person with COPD is looking to gain or lose weight, they should discuss the necessary dietary and exercise requirements with their healthcare team.

COPD and exercise

According to a 2016 review, exercise can improve muscle function and exercise tolerance in people with COPD.

Another 2016 study found that exercise and dietary restriction provided additional benefits for participants who had COPD and obesity. These benefits included:

- improved weight
- improved exercise tolerance
- improved health status

People with COPD who have underweight or have PCS may also benefit from regular exercise.

If someone with COPD wishes to take up exercise, they should discuss this with their healthcare team.

COPD: Exercise & Activity Guidelines

The benefits and types of physical activity for people with chronic obstructive pulmonary disease (COPD) are presented. Pulmonary rehabilitation might be needed.

Pulmonary rehabilitation

Pulmonary rehabilitation is a program that can help you learn how to breathe easier and improve your quality of life. It includes breathing retraining, exercise training, education, and counseling.

Why should I exercise?

Regular exercise has many benefits. Exercise, especially aerobic exercise, can:

- Improve your circulation and help the body better use oxygen

- Improve your COPD symptoms

- Build energy levels so you can do more activities without becoming tired or short of breath

- Strengthen your heart and cardiovascular system
- Increase endurance
- Lower blood pressure
- Improve muscle tone and strength; improve balance and joint flexibility
- Strengthen bones
- Help reduce body fat and help you reach a healthy weight
- Help reduce stress, tension, anxiety, and depression
- Boost self-image and self-esteem; make you look fit and feel healthy
- Improve sleep

- Make you feel more relaxed and rested

Talk to your healthcare provider first

Always check with your healthcare provider before starting an exercise program. Your healthcare provider can help you find a program that matches your level of fitness and physical condition.

Here are some questions to ask:

- How much exercise can I do each day?
- How often can I exercise each week?
- What type of exercise should I do?
- What type of activities should I avoid?
- Should I take my medicine at a certain time around my exercise schedule?

What type of exercise is best?

Exercise can be divided into 3 basic types:

1. Stretching: Slow lengthening of the muscles. Stretching the arms and legs before and after exercising helps prepare the muscles for activity and helps prevent injury and muscle strain. Regular stretching also increases your range of motion and flexibility.

2. Cardiovascular or aerobic: Steady physical activity using large muscle groups. This type of exercise strengthens the heart and lungs, and improves the body's ability to use oxygen. Over time, aerobic exercise can help decrease your heart rate and blood pressure, and improve your breathing (since your heart won't have to work as hard during exercise). Aerobic exercises include: walking, jogging, jumping rope,

bicycling (stationary or outdoor), cross-country skiing, skating, rowing, and low-impact aerobics or water aerobics.

3. Strengthening: Repeated muscle contractions (tightening) until the muscle becomes tired. Strengthening exercises for the upper body are especially helpful for people with COPD, as they help increase the strength of your respiratory muscles.

How often should I exercise?

The frequency of an exercise program is how often you exercise. In general, to achieve maximum benefits, you should gradually work up to an exercise session lasting 20 to 30 minutes, at least 3 to 4 times a week. Exercising every other day will help you keep a regular exercise schedule.

What should I include in my program?

Every exercise session should include a warm-up, conditioning phase, and a cool down. The warm-up helps your body adjust slowly from rest to exercise. A warm-up reduces the stress on your heart and muscles, slowly increases your breathing, circulation (heart rate), and body temperature. It also helps improve flexibility and reduce muscle soreness.

The best warm-up includes stretching, range of motion activities, and beginning of the activity at a low intensity level.

The conditioning phase follows the warm-up. During this phase, the benefits of exercise are gained and calories are burned. During the conditioning phase, you should monitor the intensity of the activity. The intensity is how hard you are exercising, which can be measured by checking your heart rate. Your healthcare provider can give you more information on monitoring your heart rate.

Over time, you can work on increasing the duration of the activity. The duration is how long you exercise during one session.

The cool-down phase is the last phase of your exercise session. It allows your body to gradually recover from the conditioning phase. Your heart rate and blood pressure will return to near resting values. Cool-down does not mean to sit down. In fact, do not sit, stand still, or lie down right after exercise. This might cause you to feel dizzy, lightheaded, or have heart palpitations (fluttering in your chest).

The best cool-down is to slowly decrease the intensity of your activity. You might also do some of the same stretching activities you did in the warm-up phase.

Rated Perceived Exertion (RPE) Scale

The RPE scale is used to measure the intensity of your exercise. The RPE scale runs from 0-10. The numbers below relate to phrases used to rate how easy or difficult you find an activity. For example, 0 (nothing at all) would be how you feel when sitting in a chair; 10 (very, very heavy) is how you feel at the end of an exercise stress test or after a very difficult activity.

0 - Nothing at all

0.5 - Just noticeable

1 - Very light

2 - Light

3 - Moderate

4 - Somewhat heavy

5 - Heavy

6

7 - Very heavy

8

9

10 -Very, very heavy

In most cases, you should exercise at a level that feels 3 (moderate) to 4 (somewhat heavy). When using this rating scale, remember to include feelings of shortness of breath, as well as how tired you feel in your legs and overall.

General exercise guidelines

- Gradually increase your activity level, especially if you have not been exercising regularly.

- Remember to have fun. Choose an activity you enjoy. Exercising should be fun and not a chore. You'll be more likely to stick with an exercise program if you enjoy the activity. Here are some questions you can think about before choosing a routine:

o What physical activities do I enjoy?

- Do I prefer group or individual activities?
- What programs best fit my schedule?
- Do I have physical conditions that limit my choice of exercise?
- What goals do I have in mind? (losing weight, strengthening muscles, or improving flexibility, for example)

- Wait at least 1½ hours after eating a meal before exercising.
- When drinking liquids during exercise, remember to follow your fluid restriction guidelines.
- Dress for the weather conditions and wear protective footwear.

- Take time to include a five-minute warm-up, including stretching exercises, before any aerobic activity and include a five- to 10-minute cool down after the activity. Stretching can be done while standing or sitting.

- Schedule exercise into your daily routine. Plan to exercise at the same time every day (such as in the mornings when you have more energy). Add a variety of exercises so you do not get bored.

- Exercise at a steady pace. Keep a pace that allows you to still talk during the activity.

- Exercise does not have to put a strain on your wallet. Avoid buying expensive equipment or health club memberships unless you are certain you will use them regularly.

- Stick with it. If you exercise regularly, it will soon become part of your lifestyle. Make exercise a lifetime commitment. Finding an exercise "buddy" will also help you stay motivated.

- Keep an exercise record.

Breathing during activity

Always breathe slowly to save your breath. Inhale through your nose, keeping your mouth closed. This warms and moisturizes the air you breathe and at the same time filters it. Exhale through pursed lips.

- Breathe out slowly and gently through pursed lips. This permits more complete lung action when the oxygen you inhale is exchanged for the carbon dioxide you exhale.

- Try to inhale for two seconds and exhale for four seconds. You might find slightly shorter or longer periods are more natural for you. If so, just try to breathe out twice as long as you breathe in.

- Exercise will not harm your lungs. When you experience shortness of breath during an activity, this is an indication that your body needs more oxygen. If you slow your rate of breathing and concentrate on exhaling through pursed lips, you will restore oxygen to your system more rapidly.

Walking guidelines

- Start with a short walk. See how far you can go before you become breathless. Stop and rest whenever you are short of breath.

- Count the number of steps you take while you inhale. Then exhale for twice as many steps. For example, if you inhale while taking two steps, exhale through pursed lips while taking the next four steps. Learn to walk so breathing in and exhaling out will become a habit once you find a comfortable breathing rate.

- Try to increase your walking distance. If you can set specific goals, you'll find you can go farther every day. Many people have found that an increase of 10 feet a day is a good goal.

- Set reasonable goals. Don't walk so far that you can't get back to your starting point without difficulty breathing. Remember, if you are short of breath after limited walking, stop and rest.

• Never overdo it. Always stop and rest for two or three minutes when you start to become short of breath.

Stair climbing

• Hold the handrail lightly to keep your balance and to help yourself climb.

• Take your time.

• Step up while exhaling or breathing out with pursed lips. Place your whole foot flat on each step. Go up two steps with each exhalation.

• Inhale or breathe in while taking a rest before the next step.

• Going downstairs is much easier. Hold the handrail and place each foot flat on the step. Count the number of steps you take while inhaling, and take twice as many steps while exhaling.

COPD Diet

Nutritional recommendations can play a role in chronic obstructive pulmonary disease (COPD) management. Diet can keep you at a healthy body weight; being overweight can worsen breathing, while being underweight a possible result of severe disease.

Nutrient-rich foods like fruits and vegetables are recommended, while highly processed foods or deep-fried and breaded items should be avoided.

Benefits

COPD is a lung disease that causes a number of symptoms, including dyspnea (shortness of breath) and fatigue due to airway inflammation and narrowing.

There are a variety of benefits when it comes to following nutritional recommendations in COPD. Weight control, keeping your immune system healthy, helping your lungs heal from damage, maintaining your energy, and avoiding inflammation are among the ways your diet can enhance your health when you have this disease.

These effects won't reverse the condition, but they can help keep it from getting worse.

Weight Control

Weight is complicated when it comes to COPD. Obesity is considered a COPD risk factor. And being overweight places a high demand on your heart and lungs, making you short of breath and worsening your COPD symptoms.

But malnutrition and being underweight can pose a major problem in COPD too. Chronic disease puts increased demands on your body, robbing your body of nutrients. And, a lack of nutrients makes it even harder for you to heal from the recurrent lung damage inherent with COPD.

This means that weight control is something you need to be serious about. Regularly weighing yourself can help you get back on track quickly if you veer away from your ideal weight range. Strategic diet choices, of course, can help you stay on track.

Strengthening Your Immune System

Any infection, especially a respiratory one, can make it difficult to breathe and can lead to a COPD exacerbation.

When you have COPD, a pulmonary infection has a more severe impact on your already impaired lungs. And COPD itself results in a diminished ability to avoid infections through protective mechanisms like coughing.

Getting adequate nutrients like protein, vitamin C, and vitamin D through diet can help your immune system fight off infections.

Healing From Damage

Recurrent lung damage is the core problem in COPD. When your body is injured, it needs to heal. Nutrients like vitamin E and vitamin K help your body repair itself.

Maintaining Energy

COPD leads to low energy. You need to consume carbohydrates to fuel yourself.

Iodine, an essential mineral, helps your body make thyroid hormone to regulate your energy metabolism. Your body also needs adequate vitamin B12 and iron to keep your oxygen-carrying red blood cells healthy.

Avoiding Inflammation

Inflammation plays a major role in COPD. Experts recommend a diet rich in antioxidants such as plant-based foods and omega-3 fatty acid-rich seafood to help combat excessive inflammation.

Research also suggests that artificial preservatives may induce an inflammatory response that promotes diseases such as COPD, so they should be avoided.

How does diet affect COPD?

A healthful diet can help prevent or manage some of the adverse health effects of COPD, a lung condition characterized by airflow limitation that makes it hard to breathe.

According to reviews in 2015 and 2019, a healthful, well-balanced diet can have the following beneficial health effects in people with COPD:

- reducing inflammation
- maintaining and improving muscle strength
- improving lung function
- lowering metabolic and heart disease risk

How It Works

A COPD diet plan is fairly flexible and can include many foods that you like to eat. General guidelines include:

- Avoiding allergy and asthma triggers
- Eliminating (or at least minimizing) processed foods
- Including fruits, vegetables, beans, nuts, dairy, lean meats, and seafood

You can follow a vegetarian or vegan diet if you want to, but you will need to make sure that you get enough fat and protein by eating things like avocados and healthy oils.

Duration

A COPD diet is meant to be followed for a lifetime. This is a chronic, incurable disease, and following these diet guidelines consistently can help you manage symptoms along the way.

What to Eat

Research suggests that a balanced diet rich in antioxidants and anti-inflammatory foods may help prevent and manage COPD.

The best diet for someone with COPD often depends on the person's weight and lifestyle. Below are some general tips on foods to eat and foods to avoid.

Foods to eat

The American Lung Association recommend the following types of food for people who have COPD:

Complex carbohydrates

Complex carbohydrates contain long chains of sugar molecules. The body takes time to break down these molecules. As such, complex carbohydrates provide a relatively sustained release of energy.

Foods that contain complex carbohydrates include:

- fresh fruit and starchy vegetables
- whole grains
- whole grain bread and pasta
- beans and lentils

If a person with COPD wants to gain weight, eating a variety of complex carbohydrates alongside healthful sources of fat and protein can help.

Alternatively, if a person with COPD has extra body fat to lose, replacing refined carbohydrate sources with complex carbs, protein, and healthful fat can promote weight loss.

Fiber-rich foods

According to the American Lung Association, a person with COPD should aim for around 20–30 grams of fiber each day. Foods that contain a good amount of fiber include:

- beans and lentils
- fruits and vegetables

- nuts and seeds
- whole grains, such as oats
- vegetables

Protein

A study in the International Journal of Chronic Obstructive Pulmonary Disease found that people in Vietnam with COPD had increased protein needs. Including protein-rich foods at meals and snacks may help with improving nutritional status and quality of life.

Foods that are high in protein include:

- meat and poultry
- fish
- eggs

- nuts and seeds
- legumes
- tofu
- cheese
- milk

Protein sources can help increase muscle mass and help people gain weight if needed. Alternatively, adding high-quality protein sources to meals and snacks or swapping refined carbohydrate sources with healthful proteins may promote weight loss.

Mono and polyunsaturated fats

Mono and polyunsaturated fats are healthful fats that can help lower a person's cholesterol. Some foods that contain these fats include:

- certain vegetable oils, such as olive oil and avocado oil
- certain fish, including salmon
- nuts and seeds
- avocados

According to the American Lung Association, a person with COPD who is looking to gain weight should try adding these fats to meals. If they are looking to lose weight, they should limit their intake of all fats, including mono and polyunsaturated fats.

Foods to avoid

The American Lung Association recommend that people with COPD avoid or limit the following food types:

Simple carbohydrates

Simple carbohydrates provide fewer nutrients than complex carbohydrates. Foods consisting of simple carbohydrates include:

- table sugar
- chocolate and candy
- cakes and other sugary desserts
- sugary drinks
- processed foods
- white bread and pasta

Unhealthful fats

Many high-fat foods are nutritious, and people can include them in a healthful diet. However, many highly processed foods are high-fat, and people with COPD should avoid or limit them to promote overall health.

People with COPD must avoid or limit the following high-fat foods:

- fast food
- bacon and other processed meats
- fried foods
- sugary pastries
- margarine
- ice cream

Recommended Timing

Small, frequent calorie-dense meals can help you meet your caloric needs more efficiently if you are having a hard time keeping weight on. Small meals can also help you feel less full or bloated, making it more comfortable to breathe deeply.

Cooking Tips

You might enjoy keeping track of calories, reading nutrition labels, and coming up with new recipes. But not everyone wants to focus so much on every dietary detail or spend time working on creating a meal plan.

If you prefer to follow specific instructions for a personalized menu, talk to your doctor about getting a consultation with a nutritionist or a dietitian. You can get recipes or guidelines from a professional and ask questions about how to modify dishes to your preferences and for your disease.

Sometimes, a person with COPD may experience low energy levels and may not feel up to cooking. In these instances, a person may want to consider the following options:

- Quick meals: Some healthful recipes take less than 30 minutes to prepare and cook. Buying pre-cut vegetables can reduce meal preparation times further.

- Crock-Pot: With crock-pot recipes, a person can leave all the ingredients to cook over several hours.

- Leftovers: When making meals, a person may consider cooking more than they need so they can have food the next day.

- Batch cook: On days when a person with COPD may be feeling less fatigued, they may consider batch cooking meals to keep in the freezer.

Cooking guidelines to keep in mind include:

- Use salt in moderation: This is especially important if you have high blood pressure or edema (swelling of the feet or legs). Edema is a late-stage complication of COPD.

- Use fresh herbs to add natural flavor, which can reduce your reliance on salt.

- Use natural sweeteners like honey, ginger, or cinnamon instead of sugar. Excess sugar can increase the risk of edema.

Modifications

One of the most important dietary guidelines to keep in mind when you have COPD is avoiding foods that may trigger an allergic reaction or an asthma attack.

Allergies and asthma attacks can cause severe, sudden shortness of breath. Anything that triggers a bout of breathing problems can be life-threatening for you when you already have COPD.

Common food triggers include dairy products, eggs, nuts, or soybeans.

You don't need to avoid an allergen (a substance that causes an allergic reaction) if it doesn't cause you to have symptoms, but try to be observant about patterns and trends that exacerbate your symptoms.

If you notice that certain foods affect your breathing, it's important to be vigilant about avoiding them.

Considerations

The basics of a COPD diet are healthy guidelines for everyone. Because of your COPD, however, there are some additional things you should keep in mind when working to follow your eating plan.

General Nutrition

Don't assume that you are vitamin deficient. If you and your doctor are concerned that you could be low in a nutrient like iron or vitamin D, for example, get tested first before you rush to take supplements.

If you find out that you are low in certain nutrients and can't consume enough, you can discuss supplements with your medical team. Vitamins or protein drinks may be the only way for you to get the nutrients your body needs if it's too difficult for you to consume an adequate diet.

Safety

Your tendency to cough when you have COPD could place you at risk of choking when you eat or drink. Be sure to give yourself ample time to consume your food and liquids carefully. Avoid talking while you are eating and drinking so you can reduce your risk of choking.

Shortness of breath can be a problem when eating too. Pace yourself and stick to foods that are not difficult for you to chew and swallow.

If you are on continuous oxygen therapy, make sure you use it while you eat. Since your body requires energy to eat and digest food, you will need to keep breathing in your supplemental oxygen to help you get through your meals.

Tips for eating

Some people with COPD may experience a lack of appetite due to breathing difficulties and general chest discomfort. Breathing difficulties also increase the physical effort required for eating, and this can make it difficult for a person to finish meals.

Below are some tips that may help improve a person's appetite and energy levels, or ease the effort required for eating.

- Eating smaller meals: Instead of eating three large meals a day, it may be helpful to aim to eat four to six smaller meals. This should reduce stomach fullness and associated pressure on the lungs.

- Eating the main meal earlier: A person may find that they have more energy throughout the day if they eat their main meal earlier in the day.

- Drinks: A 2019 review found that readily available high-protein, high-energy drinks can help boost nutrition in people unable to tolerate high volumes of food.

COPD DIET RECIPES

The following recipes are COPD diet-friendly while also being a treat to the taste buds. Try some of these COPD diet recipes to manage your symptoms.

Grilled Chicken and Tomato Salad

Prepartion time

20 minutes

Ingredients:

- 4 skinless, boneless chicken breast halves (6-ounce pieces)
- 5 cups of arugula salad mix
- 1 cup cherry tomatoes, halves

- ¼ cup thinly sliced red onion
- ¼ cup olive oil and vinegar salad dressing, divided
- 10 pitted and chopped Kalamata olives
- ½ cup goat cheese crumbles
- ¼ teaspoon salt
- ¼ teaspoon black pepper
- Cooking spray

Instructions

1. Heat grill pan to medium-high heat, spray pan with cooking spray when heated.
2. Season chicken with salt and pepper.

3. Place chicken on grill pan and cook for 6 minutes on each side until cooked.

4. Combine arugula, onion, tomatoes, olives, 3 tablespoons of olive oil and vinegar dressing; toss.

5. Divide salad onto four plates, top salad with 2 tablespoons of goat cheese crumbles.

6. Brush chicken with 1 tablespoon of olive oil/vinegar dressing, cut chicken into slices.

7. Divide chicken on top of the salad plates equally.

Quinoa Black Bean Salad

Prepartion time

20 minutes

Ingredients:

- 1/3 cup quinoa
- 1 can black beans (15 ounces), rinsed and drained
- 1 cup water
- 4 teaspoons fresh lime juice
- 1 teaspoon olive oil
- 1 tablespoon fresh minced cilantro
- 2 cups diced tomatoes
- 1 cup diced bell pepper
- 2 teaspoons minced jalapeno chilies

- 2 tablespoons minced scallions
- ¼ teaspoon cumin
- salt and black pepper

Instructions

1. Bring quinoa and water to a boil in a medium saucepan, reduce heat to low, cover pan and simmer for 15 minutes or until most of the water has been absorbed/tender.

2. Allow quinoa to cool.

3. Combine oil, lime juice, cumin, coriander, cilantro and scallions in a large bowl.

4. Add tomatoes, peppers, chilies and beans into the same large bowl. Stir.

5. Add cooled quinoa to a large bowl. Stir.

6. Serve cold.

Salmon with a Side Salad of Tomatoes, Oranges, and Olives

Prepartion time

30 minutes

Ingredients:

- 4 pieces of skinless salmon fillets
- 2 tablespoons olive oil

- 1 navel orange, remove peel, pith, and cut into segments
- 2 small beefsteak tomatoes, cut into wedges
- ½ cup fresh cilantro sprigs (with the stem)
- ¼ cup pitted green olives, cut into halves
- Salt and black pepper

Instructions

1. Heat 1 tablespoon of olive oil in a skillet on medium-high heat.

2. Season salmon with ½ teaspoon of salt and ¼ teaspoon of pepper.

3. Cook salmon in skillet for 4-5 minutes per side, until opaque throughout and golden brown.

4. Gently add tomatoes, olives, cilantro, orange pieces, 1 tablespoon of olive oil, and ¼ teaspoon of salt, ¼ teaspoon of pepper.

5. Serve salmon with the side salad.

Fruit Salad with Yogurt

Prepartion time

10 minutes

Ingredients:

- 1 pint fresh strawberries sliced into halves or quarters
- 1 pound seedless green grapes cut into halves
- 3 bananas, peeled and sliced into coins

- 1 container of vanilla yogurt (8 ounces)

Instructions

1. Mix strawberries, bananas, grapes and vanilla yogurt in a large bowl.

Super Shake

Prepartion time

5 minutes

Ingredients:

- 1 cup whole milk
- 1 cup ice cream (1-2 scoops)

- 1 package Carnation Instant Breakfast

Instructions

1. Pour all ingredients into a blender.

2. Mix well.

Chocolate Peanut Butter Shake

Prepartion time

5 minutes

Ingredients:

- 1/2 cup heavy whipping cream

- 3 tablespoons creamy peanut butter

- 3 tablespoons chocolate syrup
- 1-1/2 cups chocolate ice cream

Instructions

1. Pour all ingredients into a blender.
2. Mix well.

Super Pudding

Prepartion time

5 minutes

Ingredients:

- 2 cups whole milk

- 2 tablespoons vegetable oil
- 1 package instant pudding
- 3/4 cup non-fat, dry milk powder

Instructions

1. Blend milk and oil.
2. Add pudding mix and mix well.
3. Pour into dishes (1/2 cup servings).

Great Grape Slush

Prepartion time

5 minutes

Ingredients:

- 2 grape juice bars
- 1/2 cup grape juice or 7-up
- 2 tablespoons corn syrup
- 1 tablespoon corn oil

Instructions

1. Pour all ingredients into a blender.
2. Mix well.

Hard-Boiled Eggs

Prepartion time

20 minutes

Ingredients

- 1 carton of eggs

Instructions:

1. We recommend cooking the eggs in a pot covered with cold water
2. Bring to a boil over medium-high heat and then cover
3. Remove from heat and let sit for about 12 minutes
4. Drain the water, cool in a bowl of ice water (or the fridge) and peel when the eggs have cooled down

5. Keep the egg carton to store the boiled eggs afterwards

Cheese

Prepartion time

17 minutes

Ingredients

- 2 tbsps olive oil
- 1 cup scallions, sliced
- 1 celery stalk, diced

- Salt & pepper to taste
- 1 cup Arborio rice
- ½ cup balsamic vinegar (or natural grape juice)
- 4 ½ cups chicken broth
- 1 (5-oz) package of baby spinach, chopped
- 2 cups fresh peas
- 1 cup grated parmesan
- 2 ounces sliced prosciutto (optional)

Instructions:

1. Heat olive oil in a saucepan over medium heat, add scallions, diced celery, and salt and pepper to taste.

2. Cook until all veggies are tender.

3. Add in rice & cook for about 2 minutes.

4. Add in 2 ½ chicken broth, only ½ cup at a time

5. Add in spinach, peas and cook.

6. Over the next 10 minutes add in remaining broth until rice is tender.

7. Add prosciutto and Parmesan to taste

Avocados

Prepartion time

10 minutes

Ingredients

- Avocado
- Radish
- Watermelon
- Feta, mint & chives (optional)

Instructions:

1. Chop up equal parts watermelon, avocado and radish.
2. Top with feta, mint and chives and toss

Walnuts

Prepartion time

12 minutes

Instructions

- 1 cup raw walnut halves
- 2 tbsps maple syrup
- 1/8 tsp salt

Instructions:

1. Add all to a medium heat skillet.
2. Toss and stir until evaporated
3. Pour onto wax paper and let cool

Salmon

Prepartion time

5 minutes

Ingredients

- 2 cans of boneless, skinless salmon, drained
- 3 hard-boiled eggs, peeled and chopped
- 1/3 cup sweet onion, chopped (to your liking)
- ½ cup of cucumber, chopped
- 1/3 cup green onion, chopped
- ¼ cup fresh dill, chopped
- 1/3 cup greek yogurt, low fat

- 2 tbsps mayonnaise (we recommend olive oil mayonnaise)
- Salt & pepper to taste

Instructions:

1. In a medium bowl, combine all the ingredients together
2. Add salt & pepper to taste

Fruit Smoothies

Prepartion time

5 minutes

Ingredients

- 1 cup milk
- ½ cup frozen strawberries
- ½ banana

Instructions:

1. Combine all in the blender and blend to your consistency.

Oatmeal

Prepartion time

7 minutes

Ingredients

- 1 cup rolled oats
- 2 cups low fat milk
- 1 banana, mashed
- ½ tsp cinnamon (exclude if you wish)
- Salt as needed

Instructions:

1. Add all ingredients to a small saucepan and turn the heat to medium-high.

2. Once to a boil, turn the head down to low and continually stir for about 3-5 minutes.

3. When oatmeal is at a desired consistency, remove from heat and serve immediately

Popcorn

Prepartion time

15 minutes

Instructions

- Brown paper bag

- ¼ cup popcorn kernels

Instructions:

1. Pour the kernels into the bag and fold the top of the bag over so popcorn doesn't spill out

2. Microwave for about 2 minutes (for a 1000-watt microwave), or until there is a few seconds (about 3) in between popping

3. Either turn off the microwave and let sit, or take the bag out carefully.

Peanut Butter/Banana Smoothie

Prepartion time

10 minutes

Ingredients

- 1 banana, cut into 1-inch slices
- ¼ cup of peanut butter
- ¼ cup of almond milk
- 2 tbsp of non-fat vanilla yogurt
- 4 ice cubes, more for a thicker smoothie

Instructions

1. Add ice cubes to a blender and blend on pulse until broken up.

2. Add banana slices and blend until smooth.

3. Add the peanut butter, yogurt, and almond milk and blend until smooth.

4. Serve!

Ricotta Balls with Basil

Prepartion time

31 minutes

Ingredients

- 250 g ricotta
- 2 tablespoons flour
- 1 egg, separated
- Freshly ground pepper
- 15 g fresh basil, finely chopped
- 1 tablespoon chives, finely chopped
- 3 slices of stale white bread

Instructions

1. Mix the ricotta in a bowl with the flour, egg yolk, 1 teaspoon salt and freshly ground pepper.

2. Stir the basil, chives and orange peel through the mixture.

3. Divide the mixture into 20 equal portions and shape them into balls with wet hands.

4. Let the balls rest for a while.

5. Grind the bread slices into fine bread crumbs with the food processor and mix with the olive oil.

6. Pour the mixture into a deep dish.

7. Briefly beat the egg white in another deep dish.

8. Preheat the AirFryer to 200°C.

9. Carefully coat the ricotta balls in the egg white and then in the bread crumbs.

10. Put 10 balls in the basket and slide the basket into the AirFryer.

11. Set the timer to 8 minutes.

12. Bake the balls until golden brown.

13. Bake the rest of the balls in the same way.

14. Serve the ricotta balls in a platter.

Ginger Turmeric Tea

Prepartion time

10 minutes

INGREDIENTS

- 2 inch ginger root washed thinly sliced
- 2 inch turmeric root washed thinly sliced
- ½ a lemon sliced plus more for serving
- 6 cups filtered water

- Honey optional
- ⅛ teaspoon black pepper optional
- ½ tablespoon coconut oil optional

INSTRUCTIONS

1. Place the sliced ginger, turmeric and lemon in a small saucepan.

2. Add the filtered water.

3. Bring the mixture to a boil, then simmer for 5-10 minutes to deepend the color.

4. Strain and serve immediately with honey, if desired.

Pineapple pear juice

Prepartion time

5 minutes

Ingredients

- 1/2 pineapple skin removed and diced
- 1 pear

Instructions

1. Juice the pineapple and pear, enjoy!

Fresh Fruit Salad

Prepartion time

15 minutes

Ingredients

- 2 cups diced fresh pineapple
- 1 pound strawberries, hulled and sliced
- ½ pint blackberries, halved
- 4 ripe kiwis, peeled, halved and sliced
- 1 cup Lime Yogurt Fruit Salad Dressing (optional; see associated recipe)

Instructions

1. Combine pineapple, strawberries, blackberries and kiwi in a large bowl.

2. Serve with yogurt dressing, if desired.

Cool Grape

Prepartion time

5 minutes

Ingredients

- 100 g white grapes
- ¼ pineapple, peeled and in chunks
- crushed ice (from 8 ice cubes)

Instructions

1. Put the grapes and pineapple in the blender and blend until smooth.

2. Pour over crushed ice and serve immediately.

Carrot and Ginger Juice with Lime

Prepartion time

5 minutes

Ingredients

- 3-4 carrots
- 1 cm fresh ginger
- 1/2 lime

Instructions

1. Peel the carrots and the ginger using a vegetable peeler.

2. Place the carrot and ginger in the juicer (speed 2).

3. Serve immediately with lime juice to taste.

4. Carrot and Ginger Juice with Lime | Philips Chef Recipes

Roasted Spring Vegetables With Arugula Pesto

Preparation time

40 minutes

INGREDIENTS

- 4 cups baby or new potatoes, 1 to 2 inches in diameter, halved or quartered depending on size
- 5 teaspoons extra-virgin olive oil, divided
- 4 cups peeled baby carrots
- 1 bunch asparagus, trimmed and cut into thirds
- 1/2 teaspoon salt
- 1/2 cup baby arugula, for garnish
- 1 clove garlic, peeled
- 5 cups baby arugula
- 1/2 cup finely shredded Asiago cheese
- 1/4 cup toasted pine nuts, (see Tip)
- 1/4 cup extra-virgin olive oil
- 1/4 teaspoon salt

INSTRUCTIONS

1. To prepare vegetables: Position rack in upper and lower thirds of oven; preheat to 425°F.

2. Toss potatoes with 2 teaspoons oil in a large bowl and spread on a large baking sheet.

3. Roast in the lower third of the oven for 5 minutes.

4. Meanwhile, toss carrots with 2 teaspoons oil in the bowl and spread on another large baking sheet.

5. After the potatoes have roasted for 5 minutes, place the carrots in the upper third of the oven and roast potatoes and carrots for 15 minutes.

6. Toss asparagus with the remaining 1 teaspoon oil in the bowl.

7. Add to the pan with the potatoes, toss to combine and return to the oven.

8. Continue roasting until all the vegetables are tender and starting to brown, 8 to 10 minutes more.

9. To prepare pesto: Meanwhile, drop garlic through the feed tube of food processor with the motor running; process until minced.

10. Stop the machine and add arugula, cheese, pine nuts, 1/4 cup oil and 1/4 teaspoon salt.

11. Pulse and then process, scraping down the sides as necessary, until the mixture is a smooth paste.

12. Toss the roasted vegetables with 1/3 cup pesto and 1/2 teaspoon salt in the large bowl (reserve the remaining pesto for another use: refrigerate for up to 1 week or freeze).

13. Transfer to a serving dish and garnish with arugula, if desired.

Crunchy Quinoa Crusted Chicken Tenders (serves 4)

Prepartion time

20 minutes

Ingredients

- 1 1/2 cups cooked quinoa
- 1/2 cup breadcrumbs
- 1 teaspoon kosher salt
- 1/2 teaspoon garlic powder
- 1/4 teaspoon paprika
- 2 pounds chicken tenders, remove white stringy tendon
- 2 large eggs or egg whites
- olive oil

Instructions

1. Pour the quinoa onto a towel and blot to remove any excess moisture.

2. Place in a shallow bowl.

3. Add the breadcrumbs, salt, garlic powder, and paprika to the quinoa.

4. Stir to combine well.

5. In a separate shallow bowl, whisk the eggs.

6. Dip the chicken into the egg and then into the quinoa mixture pressing evenly to coat.

7. Heat a large skillet over medium high heat, add a thin coat of oil and pan sear the chicken for 4-5 minutes on each side or until quinoa is golden.

To freeze the chicken fingers before cooking

1. Place coated chicken fingers on parchment lined baking sheet and freeze for 1-2 hours.

2. Place in labeled zipper bags and freeze until to 4 months.

3. When ready to cook place a few fingers in the refrigerator for 4-12 hours to defrost and then cook.

Creamy Cole Slaw

Prepartion time

20 minutes

Ingredients

- 1 head green cabbage, finely shredded
- 2 large carrots, finely shredded
- 3/4 cup best-quality mayonnaise
- 2 tablespoons sour cream
- 2 tablespoons grated Spanish onion
- 2 tablespoons sugar, or to taste
- 2 tablespoons white vinegar
- 1 tablespoon dry mustard
- 2 teaspoons celery salt
- Salt and freshly ground pepper

Instructions

1. Combine the shredded cabbage and carrots in a large bowl.

2. Whisk together the mayonnaise, sour cream, onion, sugar, vinegar, mustard, celery salt, salt, and pepper in a medium bowl, and then add to the cabbage mixture.

3. Mix well to combine and taste for seasoning; add more salt, pepper, or sugar if desired.

Italian Pasta Salad

Prepartion time

1 hour 25 minutes

Ingredients

- 1 pound rotini pasta , uncooked
- 8 ounces fresh mozzarella cheese pearls (or chopped into pieces if you can't find pearls)
- 8 ounces salami chopped, or substitute summer sausage)
- 6 ounces black olives , sliced
- 1/2 red onion , diced
- 1 1/2 cups cherry tomatoes , halved
- 2 Tablespoons fresh parsley leaves chopped
- 1/2 cup freshly grated parmesan cheese
- pepperoncinis , sliced (optional)

For the Italian Salad Dressing (or substitute about 1 1/2 cups bottled zesty italian dressing):

- 3/4 cup olive oil
- 1/4 cup red wine vinegar
- 2 teaspoons dried parsley flakes
- 2 teaspoons dried minced onion
- 2 teaspoons fresh lemon juice
- 1 teaspoon dried basil
- 1 teaspoon dried oregano leaves
- 1 teaspoon garlic salt
- 1 teaspoon granulated sugar
- 1/4 teaspoon freshly ground black pepper

Instructions

1. Make the salad dressing by combining all ingredients.

2. Store the dressing in the refrigerator for up to 2 weeks.

3. Shake before using.

For the pasta salad:

1. Cook pasta according to package instructions.

2. Drain water and rinse pasta with cold water.

3. Allow it to cool for at least 10 minutes.

4. Add pasta to a large bowl and pour half of the salad dressing over it.

5. Toss to combine.

6. Add remaining ingredients and dressing and toss everything to combine.

7. Cover and refrigerate for 1 hour or longer, before serving.

8. Store in the fridge for up to 4-5 days.

Vanilla Bean Ice Cream with Home-made Strawberry

Prepartion time

30 minutes

Ingredients

For the Vanilla Bean Ice Cream:

- 3 cups heavy cream
- 2 vanilla beans
- 1 cup vanilla sugar regular sugar is okay too

For the Macerated Strawberries:

- 1 to 1 1/2 cups fresh strawberries washed and hulled
- Juice of 1 orange
- 1 to 2 tablespoons vanilla sugar regular sugar is fine

Instructions

For the Vanilla Bean Ice Cream:

1. Pour the heavy cream into a medium sized saucepan.

2. Place over medium low heat.

3. Take your vanilla beans and slice them down the middle all the way down the length.

4. Spread it apart as best you can and scrape the inside with a knife.

5. Take all that yummy goodness and put it in the saucepan of heavy cream.

6. Repeat with second bean, and toss both the beans in the saucepan too.

7. Now let the cream heat up until it starts to bubble all around the outside edge of the saucepan.

8. Do not let it reach full boil. You just want that slight bubbling.

9. Take it off the heat and drop in the sugar.

10. Stir until it dissolves.

11. Now allow it to cool down.

12. Place in the fridge overnight, (you can do it for a shorter time but the vanilla taste will be more subtle) covered.

13. Remove from the fridge and pull out the large pieces of beans.

14. Pop in your ice cream maker and allow to spin for 10 to 15 minutes.

15. This is a steeped cream base so it will not double up like some ice cream bases. It yields less but is far more creamy.

16. Pop the ice cream attachment in the freezer overnight, you could do it for less time but it will not be as firm.

17. Remove from freezer when ready to serve.

18. Since this is a creamy base it tends to melt quicker so keep that in mind when scooping.

19. Serve solo or with berries.

For the Strawberry Topping:

1. Hull and slice up your strawberries into a medium sized bowl, or container.

2. Cut an orange in half. Juice it over top of the strawberries.

3. Discard the orange.

4. Cover and place in the fridge for about 2 to 4 hours. The longer they sit the softer they become.

5. Remove and sprinkle some sugar over top.

Putting it all together:

1. Scoop out some ice cream, working quickly.

2. Scoop some strawberries over top.

3. You can top with anything else you like, I threw pistachios over top of mine, but you could use walnuts or almonds or chocolate pieces.

4. Serve.

Roast Chicken with Garlic and Herb Pan Sauce

Prepartion time

1 hour 15 minutes

Ingredients

- 1 3 to 4 pound chicken, preferably organic or free-range, brought to room temperature
- 1 pinch Kosher salt (and pepper if you'd like)
- 1/3 cup olive oil
- 1 tablespoon unsalted butter

- 2 large sprigs of thyme
- 2 garlic cloves, peeled and smashed
- 1/4 cup white wine

Instructions

1. Heat the oven to 480° F.

2. Pat the chicken dry inside and out (if you want an extra crispy skin, leave the raw chicken in the fridge uncovered overnight after you've patted it dry and then bring it to room temperature).

3. Put the chicken on a board or a large platter and generously season the inside of the bird with salt and pepper if you're using it.

4. Drizzle a little olive oil in the cavity as well.

5. Drizzle the rest of the oil over the chicken, and rub it all over so that it's evenly coated.

6. Salt the chicken well all over, making sure to get into all the nooks and crannies.

7. Transfer the chicken to an enameled cast iron pan or a heavy roasting pan just big enough to hold it and put it in the oven.

8. Don't open the door for at least 45 minutes, when you can start to test it for doneness. (The chicken is cooked when you pierce the thickest part of the thigh with a sharp knife, and the juices run clear.)

9. Let the chicken rest on a carving board while you make the pan sauce.

10. To make the sauce, put the roasting pan on the stove over medium-high heat.

11. Add the butter to the drippings in the pan, and once it melts add the thyme and garlic.

12. Cook, stirring frequently, for about a minute.

13. Add the wine to the pan and scrape up all the brown bits with a wooden spoon, stirring them into the sauce.

14. Let the wine cook down for one to two minutes.

15. Add a cup of boiling water, stir well, and let the sauce reduce for about 5 minutes.

16. Taste and add more salt if necessary (if you've salted your chicken enough, this probably won't be necessary).

17. Cut the chicken into pieces and serve with the warm pan sauce in a bowl nearby for dipping.

Mixed Berry Smoothies

Prepartion time

5 minutes

Ingredients

- 1/4 cup water
- 1 cup raspberries
- 1 cup strawberries
- 1/2 cup blueberries
- 1/2 cup cottage cheese
- 1 handful of ice cubes (See Kelly's Notes)
- 2 teaspoons honey or agave nectar

Instructions

1. Add all of the ingredients to the blender in the order in which they are listed.

2. Blend until smooth and pourable.

3. Taste and adjust the sweetness by adding more honey or agave nectar as desired.

Creamy Spinach Dip

Prepartion time

5 minutes

INGREDIENTS

- 1 small shallot, peeled
- 1 5-ounce can water chestnuts, rinsed
- 1/2 cup reduced-fat cream cheese, Neufchâtel
- 1/2 cup low-fat cottage cheese
- 1/4 cup nonfat plain yogurt

- 1 tablespoon lemon juice
- 1/2 teaspoon salt
- 6 ounces baby spinach
- 2 tablespoons chopped fresh chives
- freshly ground pepper, to taste

INSTRUCTIONS

1. Pulse shallot and water chestnuts in a food processor until coarsely chopped.

2. Add cream cheese, cottage cheese, yogurt, lemon juice, salt and pepper and pulse until just combined.

3. Add spinach and chives and pulse until incorporated.

Baked Vegan Cheesecake with Berries

Prepartion time

1 hour 15 minutes

Ingredients

Crust

- 1 ½ cups (240g) plain flour or gluten-free flour blend
- ½ cup (50g) blanched almond meal / almond flour, or substitute with more flour
- ¼ cup (40g) cane sugar, or coconut sugar
- ¾ cup (180g) vegan butter, or solid refined coconut oil

Cheesecake filling

- 2 cups (260g) raw cashews*
- 1 cup (250g) firm silken tofu, also known as 'traditional tofu'**
- ½ cup (180g) any light-coloured sweetener, such as rice malt syrup or maple syrup, to taste
- ½ cup (90g) dairy free yoghurt, such as coconut, soy or almond
- ¼ cup (60g) dairy free milk, such as almond, soy or coconut
- 1 tbsp (7g) corn starch / corn flour, optional but creates a smoother cheesecake
- 2 tsp lemon juice, or apple cider vinegar***

- 2 tsp vanilla extract, or vanilla bean powder
- Pinch of any good-quality salt

To decorate

- 1 ½ cups (225g) frozen or fresh blueberries and raspberries
- ¼ cup (100g) any light-coloured sweetener, such as rice malt syrup or maple syrup, optional and to taste
- 1 tbsp (7g) corn starch / corn flour

Instructions

1. Preheat the oven to 180°C (350°F).

2. Line the bottom and sides of a spring-form or loose-bottom cake tin. I used a tall 20 cm (8-inch) cake tin.

To make the crust:

1. In a large bowl or food processor, mix all the crust ingredients until well combined.

2. It should stick together when pinched between two fingers.

3. If the mixture is still a bit dry, add a dash of water and mix until the ingredients come together.

4. Firmly press the mixture into the bottom and sides of the lined cake tin so it's about 8 mm thick.

5. Bake the crust for 15 minutes or until slightly golden and it's dry to the touch.

6. Set aside.

To make the filling:

1. Add all ingredients to a blender and blend until there are no lumps.

2. Taste and adjust the level of sweetness and sourness, if needed.

3. Pour the cheesecake filling into the crust.

4. Tap the cheesecake firmly on the counter a few times to remove any air bubbles.

5. Baking the cheesecake:

6. Bake the cheesecake for 45-50 minutes, just before the filling sets. If the crust is browning too quickly, cover the cheesecake with a metal tray. The cheesecake is ready when the filling is no longer liquid and the filling still 'jiggles' in the middle.

7. Allow the cheesecake to cool in the oven with the door ajar for at least 1 hour.

8. Remove the cheesecake from the oven. Let it come to room temperature, cover it and set it aside in the fridge overnight to chill.

9. The next day, prepare the berry topping:

10. Add all or most of the berries and rest of the ingredients to a small saucepan and mix until combined.

11. Place the saucepan over medium heat and mix for 5 minutes until thickened.

12. Remove from the heat and allow it to cool.

13. Remove the cheesecake from its tin.

14. Spoon and spread the berry topping on top and top with additional berries if desired.

15. Cut and serve!

16. The cheesecake can be kept in an airtight container at room temperature for 1 day or in the fridge for up to 5 days.

EASY COLD CRAB DIP RECIPE WITH CREAM CHEESE

Prepartion time

5 minutes

INGREDIENTS

- 4 oz Cream cheese (softened)
- 3 tbsp Sour cream
- 1 tsp Lemon juice
- 1/4 tsp Old Bay seasoning (adjust more or less to taste)
- 8 oz Lump crab meat (squeezed to remove any water/moisture)
- 2 tbsp Chives (chopped)

INSTRUCTIONS

1. Blend together the cream cheese, sour cream, lemon juice, and seasoning in a blender or food processor, until smooth.

2. Fold in the crab meat and chives using a spatula. (Do this gently and don't over-mix. You want some lumps of crab throughout.)

3. Transfer to a bowl, cover in plastic wrap, and chill until ready to serve.

www.ingramcontent.com/pod-product-compliance
Ingram Content Group UK Ltd.
Pitfield, Milton Keynes, MK11 3LW, UK
UKHW022003190726
13853UKWH00004B/1705

9 798539 876005